D1634697

Follicular Lymphoma:
Fast Focus Study Guide

JT Thomas, MD

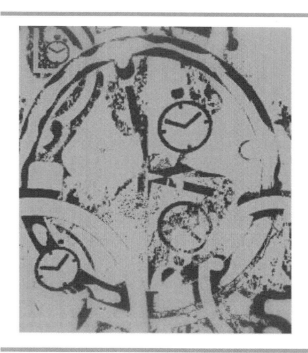

Acknowledgements

I dedicate this book to my beautiful wife and children, who I love more than all the water in all the oceans and all the seas.

CONTENTS

- This book is written to help the reader further understand Follicular Lymphoma.

- This book is written in a simple and easy to read format designed for medical students, residents and physicians who are preparing for boards.

- This book simplifies a complicated medical issue so you will remember the important details.

- You will not get caught up in the minutia. Just the facts are found in this book.

- This Fast Focus Study Guide will provide you with a practical review of the key information you need to know.

- Buy this book now if you want this quick and concise information

Follicular Lymphoma is the most common type of non-Hodgkin lymphoma.

There are approximately 15,000 cases of

Follicular Lymphoma in the US per year.

Follicular Lymphoma

-Accounts for 30-40% of lymphomas in the adult population in western countries

-Peak incidence in the 5th and 6th decade

-Immunophenotypic profile is CD 10+, CD5-, sig+

-70-80% of cases will have t(14;18)(q32;q21)

Follicular Lymphoma

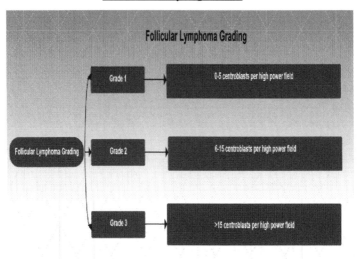

Follicular Lymphoma Grading

Follicular Lymphoma Grading

Grade 1 → 0-5 centroblasts per high power field

Grade 2 → 6-15 centroblasts per high power field

Grade 3 → >15 centroblasts per high power field

A centroblast generally refers to an activated B cell that is enlarged and proliferating. These metabolically ative B cells proliferate in the germinal center of a secondary lymphoid follicle following exposure to a follicular dendritic cell cytokines such as IL6, IL15 and BAFF

Grade 3 Follicular lymphoma accounts for < 20% of cases.

Grade 3 Follicular lymphoma can be separated

into 3A and 3B

We separate the Grade 3 Follicular lymphoma into 3A and 3B. We do this because the treatment can change.

Grade 3A follicular lymphoma is characterized by the fact that centrocytes are present.

Grade 3B Follicular lymphoma is characterized by solid sheets of centroblasts without centrocytes.

Grade 3A Follicular lymphoma is typically treated like grade 1 and grade 2 Follicular lymphoma.

Grade 3B Follicular lymphoma is usually treated like diffuse large cell B cell NHL.

Staging Follicular Lymphoma.

Stage I

Only one lymph node region is involved, or only one lymph structure is involved.

Stage II

Two or more lymph node regions or lymph node structures on the same side of the diaphragm are involved.

Stage III

Lymph node regions or structures on both sides of the diaphragm are involved

Stage IV

There is widespread involvement of a number of organs or tissues other than lymph node regions or structures, such as the bone marrow.

Flow Cytometry of Follicular Lymphoma

The flow cytometry is positive for CD20, CD10, BCL2, and BCL6. It is negative for CD 5. I remember that CD 5 differentiates Follicular lymphoma from CLL because CLL is positive for CD5.

CD 20+

CD 20+ is easy to remember because I know that this is a pan B cell marker

CD 10+

CD 10 is also known as Common Acute Lymphoblastic Leukemia Antigen (CALLA). It is a cell membrane metallopeptidase widely distributed in hematopoietic cells

BCL 6+

BCL 6 is a zinc finger transcription factor that acts as a sequence-specific repressor of transcription, and has been shown to modulate the transcription of START-dependent IL-4 responses of B cells.

BCL-2 +

Bcl-2 is an oncogene that regulates cell death (apoptosis), by either inducing (pro-apoptotic) it or inhibiting it (anti-apoptotic).

CD 5-

CD 5 is considered a good T-cell marker but is also found on IgM-secreting B cells. It is negative in Follicular lymphoma but positive in CLL

Cytogenetics

Approximately 90% of Follicular lymphoma
will be characterized by t(14;18).

Cytogenetics

Grade 1 and 2 Follicular lymphoma is more likely to have the t(14;18) than grade 3 Follicular lymphoma.

A solitary skin lesion that has characteristics of a low grade lymphoma should be evaluated for primary cutaneous follicular center cell lymphoma.

Primary cutaneous follicular center lymphoma

Grows as follicular, follicular and diffuse, or diffuse growth pattern.

Primary cutaneous follicular center lymphoma

Cells are BCL 2 negative

Primary cutaneous follicular center lymphoma

This is a type lymphoma develops from
follicular center cells

Primary cutaneous follicular center lymphoma

Develops as skin lesions on the trunk,
forehead, or scalp.

Primary cutaneous follicular center lymphoma

Most of these are not multifocal

Primary cutaneous follicular center lymphoma

Typically grows slowly

Treatment Stage I and II Follicular Lymphoma

Stage I and II disease is treated with radiation

Treatment Stage I and II Follicular Lymphoma

If there is a lymph node > 5 cm could consider combined modality treatment with both chemotherapy and radiation

Treatment Stage I and II Follicular Lymphoma

It is alright to consider the watch and wait approach

Stage III and IV

Patients with low tumor burden and no symptoms can be treated with watch and wait or rituximab

Stage III and IV

Patients with low tumor burden with symptoms can be treated with rituximab or rituximab and chemo.

Stage III and IV

Patients with high tumor burden with no symptoms can be treated watch and wait or rituximab.

Stage III and IV

Patients with high tumor burden with symptoms can be treated with chemo and rituximab

We use the GELF Criteria to determine if a patient with follicular lymphoma has high tumor burden:

- A tumor >7 cm in diameter

- Three nodes in three distinct areas, each >3 cm in diameter

- Symptomatic spleen enlargement

- Organ compression

- Ascites or pleural effusion.

GELF Criteria to determine high tumor
burden disease

Any nodal or extra nodal mass >7cm

GELF Criteria to determine high tumor
burden disease

Three or more nodal sites with diameter > 3
cm

GELF Criteria to determine high tumor burden disease

Elevated LDH

GELF Criteria to determine high tumor burden disease

Hemoglobin < 10g/dl, Absolute Neutrophil Count < 1.5 x 10(9), Platelets < 100,000

GELF Criteria to determine high tumor
burden disease

Spleen >16 cm by CT scan

GELF Criteria to determine high tumor burden disease

Organ compression

GELF Criteria to determine high tumor burden disease

Ascites or Pleural Effusion

What are the trials that helped defined

Follicular Lymphoma treatment?

The clinical trials for Follicular lymphoma treatment have defined the following:

-Watch and wait is reasonable in low tumor burden asymptomatic patients.

-Immediate Rituximab treatment is associated with improved PFS and longer time to first chemotherapy.

-Approximately 15% of patients may experience improved Quality of Life with single agent Rituximab.

Is maintenance Rituximab beneficial in
patients with Follicular Lymphoma?

Maintenance Rituximab May Improve
Survival in Follicular Lymphoma

J Natl Cancer Inst. 2009 Feb 18;101(4):248-55.

doi: 10.1093/jnci/djn478. Epub 2009 Feb 10.

Summary

In a pooled analysis of data from five clinical trials in patients with follicular lymphoma whose disease had relapsed or was resistant to treatment, those who received maintenance therapy with rituximab survived longer than those who did not receive maintenance therapy. However, this finding leaves unanswered the question of whether maintenance rituximab is superior to treatment with rituximab on relapse.

Results

In the overall analysis, a survival benefit of maintenance rituximab appeared to be restricted to patients with previously treated (that is, refractory or relapsed) follicular lymphoma; no such benefit was seen in patients who had not received previous treatment for follicular lymphoma.

Patients treated with rituximab maintenance therapy developed more severe infections and other adverse effects than patients in the control group.

Is R-Bendamustine better than R-CHOP in patients with Follicular Lymphoma?

The German trial.

This trial presented at ASH in 2009 suggests new first-line treatment option for slow-growing lymphomas.

Bendamustine Plus Rituximab Is superior in respect of Progression Free Survival and CR Rate When Compared to CHOP Plus Rituximab as First-Line Treatment of Patients with Advanced Follicular, Indolent, and Mantle Cell Lymphomas: Final Results of a Randomized Phase III Study (Study Group Indolent Lymphomas, Germany).

Is there a survival benefit from R-Bendamustine versus R-CHOP in patients with Follicular Lymphoma?

Updated findings from a large European clinical trial indicate that patients with some types of lymphoma could initially be treated with bendamustine and rituximab. The majority of patients in the trial had follicular lymphoma, and the remainder had either mantle cell or indolent (slow-growing) lymphoma.

After a median follow-up of nearly 4 years, patients who received the two-drug combination lived more than twice as long without their disease progressing (69.5 months versus 31.2 months) as patients who received the standard first line treatment, rituximab and a chemotherapy regimen CHOP or R-CHOP.

Is maintenance Rituximab in patients with high burden disease (remember the GELF criteria) initially treated with chemotherapy associated with an improved overall survival?

Rituximab maintenance for 2 years in patients with high tumor burden follicular lymphoma responding to rituximab plus chemotherapy (PRIMA): a phase 3, randomized controlled trial.

Lancet. 2011 Jan 1;377(9759):42-51. doi: 10.1016/S0140-6736(10)62175-7. Epub 2010 Dec 20.

2 years of rituximab maintenance therapy after immunochemotherapy as first-line treatment for follicular lymphoma significantly improves progression free survival.

Is maintenance Rituximab in patients with low burden disease (remember the GELF criteria) initially treated with Rituximab associated with an improved overall survival?

J Clin Oncol. 2014 Oct 1;32(28):3096-102.
doi: 10.1200/JCO.2014.56.5853. Epub 2014
Aug 25.

Rituximab extended schedule or re-treatment
trial for low-tumor burden follicular
lymphoma: eastern cooperative oncology
group protocol e4402.

The difference in time to treatment failure
between the treatment groups was not
statistically significant.

Can idealisib be used in the setting of

recurrent Follicular lymphoma?

N Engl J Med. 2014 Mar 13;370(11):1008-18.
doi: 10.1056/NEJMoa1314583. Epub 2014 Jan
22.

PI3Kδ inhibition by idelalisib in patients with
relapsed indolent lymphoma.

The overall response rate was in the range of
57%, which included a 6% complete response
rate. In the patients with Follicular
lymphoma, the overall response rate was 54%.
At a median follow-up of 9.7 months, the
estimated 1-year survival was 80%. The
overall, the median duration of response was
12.5 months. At 48 weeks, 47% of the
patients were still progression free. The
median overall survival was 20.3 months.

Is there any way to determine prognosis in

patients with Follicular lymphoma

Components of the FLIPI Score:

1. Over 60 years of age

2. Disease at stage III or IV

3. Five or more nodules or tumors detected, or more than four lymph node groups involved

4. Serum hemoglobin less than 12 g/dL

5. Elevated serum LDH

FLIPI Scores

0-1 points/Low risk. These patients have a 91 percent survival rate at 5 years from diagnosis and 71 percent at 10 years.

2 points/Intermediate risk. These patients have a 5 year survival rate of 78 percent and the ten year survival of 51 percent.

3-5 points/High risk. These patients have a 5 survival of 53 percent and a 10 year survival of 36 percent.

What do you do when a patient relapses with
Follicular lymphoma after initial treatment
with CHOP or CVP?

In that situation we would generally consider cautiously using Fludarabine based treatment when possible

When do you think about a stem cell transplant?

In Follicular lymphoma we can consider an autologous stem cell transplant.

We usually think about autologous stem cell transplants based on a trial done in 2003 where they compared autologous to allogeneic transplants. They found lower 5 year recurrence rate with the allogeneic transplant. However, this was associated with increased transplant related mortality.

Scenario 1:

The patient is elderly. He does not meet GELF criteria for high tumor burden.

You are asked to compare treating with rituximab 4 weekly doses followed by maintenance for 2 years versus watch and wait.

Based on a UK trial you know that treatment with the Rituximab significantly prolongs time to initiation of new therapy; but, 3-year overall survival (OS) was not significantly different. For that reason, patients with asymptomatic, low tumor burden follicular lymphoma, are treated with observation as the standard of care.

You are going to remember the GELF Criteria for high tumor volume

- A tumor >7 cm in diameter

- Three nodes in three distinct areas, each >3 cm in diameter

- Symptomatic spleen enlargement

- Organ compression

- Ascites or pleural effusion

You are asked about another elderly patient with Follicular lymphoma and low burden disease by GELF criteria that you have been monitoring for 4 years. This patient has obvious progressive disease in some areas and not in other areas.

The question asks about restaging with PET scan?

You want to do a PET scan because the patient is going to need a biopsy to evaluate for transformation and you will be looking for a good target which could be characterized by increased SUV radiotracer uptake.

You have an elderly patient with a 6 cm mass that is biopsy proven follicular lymphoma. The question will ask you if the patient meets criteria for increased tumor burden.

You are going to remember the GELF Criteria for high tumor volume

- A tumor >7 cm in diameter

- Three nodes in three distinct areas, each >3 cm in diameter

- Symptomatic spleen enlargement

- Organ compression

- Ascites or pleural effusion

Scenario 4

You have another elderly patient who has Follicular lymphoma. This one has stage IV disease, and is symptomatic. The question is going to ask you why you would give Bendamustine and rituximab as opposed to R-CHOP.

You are going to think the German Trial (review the next page).

The German trial.

This trial presented at ASH in 2009 suggests new first-line treatment option for slow-growing lymphomas.

Bendamustine Plus Rituximab Is superior in respect of Progression Free Survival and CR Rate When Compared to CHOP Plus Rituximab as First-Line Treatment of Patients with Advanced Follicular, Indolent, and Mantle Cell Lymphomas: Final Results of a Randomized Phase III Study by the Study Group Indolent Lymphomas, Germany.

You are asked about the difference in toxicity
of R-CHOP versus R-Bendamustine?

Patients treated with bendamustine plus rituximab had significantly lower rates of infections and of dangerous drops in white blood cells (WBC), and as a result they were much less likely to require treatment with granulocyte colony-stimulating factor to increase WBC production.

Scenario 5

Another elderly patient. He has Follicular lymphoma. The question wants to know if R-Bendamustine is associated with improved survival when compared to R-CHOP.

You are going to think about the GERMAN trial again, this time the update in 2013

You know that the R-Bendamustine is associated with less toxicity. You also know that the first report from the German trial showed an improved progression free survival as noted below However, the two-drug regimen offered superior outcomes over R-CHOP. Median progression-free survival was 54.9 months versus 34.8 months, respectively, while the complete response rate was 39.6 percent versus 30 percent.

In the update from the GERMAN trial in 2013 they found that:

Despite the improvement in progression-free survival in patients treated with bendamustine and rituximab, overall survival did not differ between the two patient groups.

Scenario 6

You have another elderly patient. This patient is treated with R-Bendamustine. You are asked which toxicity is seen more in R-Bendamustine compared to R-CHOP.

You are going to remember the report from the German Trial.

Although there was a higher incidence of mild skin reactions in patients who received bendamustine and rituximab, other major side effects were far less common, including neuropathy and neutropenia.

Scenario 7

Another patient with Stage IV disease. You treated her with 6 cycles of R-Chemo. Now you restage her and she has very little disease present.

You are asked whether maintenance rituximab is associated with an improved overall survival.

Rituximab maintenance for 2 years in patients with high tumor burden follicular lymphoma responding to rituximab plus chemotherapy (PRIMA): a phase 3, randomized controlled trial.

Lancet. 2011 Jan 1;377(9759):42-51. doi: 10.1016/S0140-6736(10)62175-7. Epub 2010 Dec 20.

2 years of rituximab maintenance therapy after immunochemotherapy as first-line treatment for follicular lymphoma significantly improves progression free survival.

The PRIMA update noted that there were benefits for maintenance rituximab but there was no evidence of improved overall survival.

Scenario 9

You have an elderly patient with Follicular lymphoma. She was treated with chemotherapy and rituximab. Several years later she has recurrence. The question will ask you what factors you should take into consideration when considering more treatment.

There are several factors that could impact your decision. Think of the GELF criteria (see next page). Also consider symptoms, response to and toxicity from prior therapy, age, performance status, patient preference, and the possible transformation to aggressive lymphoma.

You are going to remember the GELF Criteria for high tumor volume

- A tumor >7 cm in diameter

- Three nodes in three distinct areas, each >3 cm in diameter

- Symptomatic spleen enlargement

- Organ compression

- Ascites or pleural effusion

Scenario 9

You have an elderly patient. He has been previously treated for Follicular lymphoma. R-Chemo resulted in 2 years of remission, but restaging scans show evidence of recurrence. The question will ask you if you can watch and wait.

In the setting of recurrent Follicular lymphoma after previous treatment you can watch and wait if the patient is asymptomatic and does not meet GELF criteria.

Scenario 10

The patient has a diagnosis of Follicular lymphoma. She has been heavily pretreated in the past. She has symptomatic disease. You decide to give her idelalsib. The question is going to ask you the response rate to this treatment in patients who have progressed through alkylating agents and rituximab.

N Engl J Med. 2014 Mar 13;370(11):1008-18. doi: 10.1056/NEJMoa1314583. Epub 2014 Jan 22.

PI3Kδ inhibition by idelalisib in patients with relapsed indolent lymphoma.

The ORR was 57%, which included a 6% CR rate. In the subgroup of patients with FL, the ORR was 54%. Overall, the median duration of response was 12.5 months. The median PFS was 11.0 months. At 48 weeks, 47% of the patients were still progression free. The median overall survival was 20.3 months at the time of data cutoff for the published analysis. At a median follow-up of 9.7 months, the estimated 1-year survival was 80%.

What is the mechanism of idelalsib?

Idelalisib is a selective inhibitor of the PI3 Kinase Delta (PI3Kδ) isoform that plays an important role in the survival of malignant lymphocytes by interfering in the activation, proliferation, and survival of B cells.

What kind of side effects are seen with idelalisib?

Side effects include diarrhea, fatigue, nausea, cough, and fever, rash, elevated liver tests.

What were the overall response rates (ORRs) using Lenalidomide/rituximab combination in patients with untreated follicular lymphoma?

Answer: >90%

This concludes Follicular Lymphoma: Fast Focus
Study Guide

Search Amazon Kindle books to find other study
guides written by

JT Thomas, MD

Internal Medicine Study Guide

Hematology Study Guide

Medical Oncology Study Guide

Cardiology Study Guide

Multiple Myeloma Study Guide

Differential Diagnosis Study Guide

Rheumatology Study Guide

Cancer Study Guide

Printed in Great Britain
by Amazon